The No-Diet Diet

How to Enjoy Your Favorite Foods and Still Lose Weight

MICHELLE J WILLIAMS

TABLE OF CONTENTS

INTRODUCTION

Welcome to "The No-Diet Diet: How to Eat What You Love and Still Lose Weight." If you're like many people, you may be feeling frustrated and overwhelmed by the constant barrage of conflicting weight loss advice out there. But the truth is, losing weight doesn't have to be complicated or stressful. In fact, it can be simple and enjoyable if you have the right approach.

That's what this book is all about. In these pages, you'll learn how to ditch the diet mentality and embrace a healthy, sustainable approach to weight loss that works for you. Whether you're looking to lose a few pounds or make a complete lifestyle transformation, "The No-Diet Diet" has something for everyone.

Meet Sarah, a 35-year-old woman who has been struggling with her weight for as long as she can remember. Like many of us, Sarah has tried every diet under the sun, from low-carb to low-fat to juice cleanses. But no matter how hard she tried, she always seemed to end up right back where she started. Frustrated and exhausted, Sarah began to feel like she was trapped in an endless cycle of dieting and disappointment.

That is, until she discovered the "no-diet diet." With this simple yet powerful approach, Sarah was finally able to break free from the dieting mentality and embrace a healthy, sustainable lifestyle that allowed her to eat the foods she loved and still achieve her weight loss goals.

In "The No-Diet Diet," Sarah shares her story and the lessons she learned along the way. Through engaging, personal anecdotes and practical advice, she shows readers how to overcome the obstacles that have held them back in the past and adopt healthy habits that will last a lifetime.

Whether you're looking to lose a few pounds or make a complete lifestyle transformation, "The No-Diet Diet" is the ultimate guide to achieving your weight loss goals without sacrificing the foods you love. With Sarah as your guide, you'll learn how to break free from the dieting cycle and embrace a healthy, sustainable approach to weight loss that works for you.

As a registered dietitian, I understand the challenges of trying to lose weight and maintain a healthy lifestyle. That's why I've dedicated my career to helping people like Sarah find a better way.

Through my work with clients, I've discovered that the key to lasting weight loss is not about deprivation or strict rules, but about finding a healthy balance that works for you. And that's exactly what "The No-Diet Diet" is all about.

In this book, you'll learn how to:

Ditch the diet mentality and embrace a healthy, sustainable approach to weight loss

Enjoy the foods you love without feeling guilty or deprived

Make small, simple changes that add up to big results

Find your own path to weight loss success, whatever that may look like for you

I know that losing weight can be difficult, but it doesn't have to be. With "The No-Diet Diet," you'll have the tools and support you need to make lasting changes and achieve your weight loss goals for good.

One of the biggest mistakes people make when trying to lose weight is following a one-size-fits-all diet plan. But the truth is, what works for one person may not work for another. That's why in "The No-Diet Diet," I encourage readers to find their own path to weight loss success.

That means ditching the strict rules and unrealistic goals, and instead focusing on finding a healthy balance that works for you. This might mean learning to listen to your body's hunger and fullness cues, or finding ways to incorporate more physical activity into your daily routine.

Whatever your goals and needs, "The No-Diet Diet" has something for everyone. From delicious, satisfying recipes to practical tips and strategies for staying on track, this book is your ultimate guide to losing weight and keeping it off for good. You deserve to feel confident, healthy, and happy, and this book will show you how to get there.

CHAPTER ONE

Understanding the Psychology of Weight Loss

One of the biggest challenges of losing weight is the mental and emotional aspect. It's easy to get caught up in the numbers on the scale and the endless cycle of dieting and deprivation, but the key to lasting weight loss is understanding the psychology behind it.

In this chapter, we'll explore the common mental and emotional barriers that can hold you back from achieving your weight loss goals. We'll also discuss the importance of self-compassion and self-care, and how to overcome negative self-talk and build a healthy relationship with food and your body.

One of the biggest mistakes people make when trying to lose weight is focusing on external goals like a certain number on the scale or fitting into a certain size of clothes. But the truth is, lasting weight loss is not about achieving an external goal, but about finding a healthy balance that works for you.

That means learning to listen to your body's hunger and fullness cues, and making healthy choices that nourish both your body and your mind. It also means finding ways to incorporate physical activity into your daily routine, not just for the purpose of burning calories, but for the overall health benefits it provides.

Another important aspect of the psychology of weight loss is understanding the role that emotions play in our eating habits. It's common to turn to food as a coping mechanism when we're feeling stressed, anxious, or depressed. But this can lead to unhealthy eating patterns and ultimately undermine our weight loss efforts.

That's why it's important to address the emotional factors that may be contributing to your weight gain. This might involve seeking support from a therapist or counselor, finding healthy ways to manage stress, or learning to identify and address negative thought patterns.

It's also important to practice self-compassion and learn to be kind to yourself. Too often, we criticize and judge ourselves for not being thin enough or for not making progress fast enough. But this kind of negative self-talk can be damaging and ultimately hold us back from achieving our goals.

Instead, try to cultivate a sense of self-acceptance and embrace the journey of weight loss. Remember that progress is not always linear and it's okay to have setbacks along the way. By practicing self-compassion, you'll be more likely to persevere and ultimately achieve your weight loss goals.

Sarah had always struggled with her weight, and like many people, she had tried every diet under the sun in an effort to lose weight and feel better about herself. But no matter how hard she tried, she always seemed to end up right back where she started. Frustrated and exhausted,

Sarah began to feel like she was trapped in an endless cycle of dieting and disappointment.

It wasn't until Sarah began working with a registered dietitian that she began to understand the psychology behind her weight struggles. She learned that her emotional eating habits were a major contributor to her weight gain, and that by addressing these underlying issues, she could break free from the dieting cycle and find a healthy, sustainable approach to weight loss.

Sarah also learned the importance of self-compassion and self-care. Instead of criticizing herself for not being thin enough or making progress fast enough, she began to focus on the progress she had made and the small, healthy changes she was making in her life.

Through this process, Sarah was able to break free from the dieting mentality and embrace a healthy, sustainable approach to weight loss. And with the support of her registered dietitian and the techniques she learned, Sarah was able to lose weight and keep it off for good.

Sarah's story is just one example of the transformative power of understanding the psychology of weight loss. By learning to manage your emotions and cultivate a sense of self-compassion, you too can break free from the dieting cycle and achieve your weight loss goals for good.

One of the biggest misconceptions about weight loss is that it requires strict rules and deprivation. But the truth

is, lasting weight loss is not about giving up the foods you love or restricting yourself to a certain number of calories. It's about finding a healthy balance that works for you.

That's why in "The No-Diet Diet," we encourage readers to ditch the diet mentality and embrace a healthy, sustainable approach to weight loss. This means learning to listen to your body's hunger and fullness cues and making healthy choices that nourish both your body and your mind.

It also means finding ways to incorporate physical activity into your daily routine, not just for the purpose of burning calories, but for the overall health benefits it provides. And it means learning to manage your emotions and practice self-compassion, so that you can overcome the mental and emotional barriers that may be holding you back.

By adopting these healthy habits, you'll be well on your way to achieving your weight loss goals and living a healthy, sustainable lifestyle. And the best part is, you'll be able to eat the foods you love without feeling deprived or restricted.

Weight loss can be a complex and difficult process, and there are many factors that can contribute to success or challenges. Understanding the psychology of weight loss can be helpful in developing strategies for achieving and maintaining a healthy weight.

One key factor is motivation. Having a clear and strong motivation for losing weight can help you stay focused and committed to your goals. This might be a desire to improve your health, to feel more confident and self-assured, or to fit into clothing more comfortably.

Another important factor is self-regulation, which refers to your ability to manage your thoughts, emotions, and behaviors in order to reach your goals. This can be challenging when it comes to weight loss, as it often requires making changes to your diet and exercise habits, which can be difficult to sustain over time.

Mindfulness and awareness of your thoughts, feelings, and behaviors can also be helpful in weight loss efforts. This includes being aware of triggers that may lead to unhealthy eating habits or a lack of physical activity, and finding ways to cope with these challenges in a healthy way.

It can also be helpful to surround yourself with supportive people who can encourage and motivate you on your weight loss journey. This might include friends, family members, or a support group.

Ultimately, the psychology of weight loss involves understanding your own motivations, developing self-regulation skills, and finding ways to cope with challenges and setbacks. With patience, persistence, and a positive attitude, you can work towards achieving and maintaining a healthy weight.

One of the key psychological factors that can impact weight loss is self-esteem. Individuals with low self-esteem may be more prone to emotional eating, which can sabotage weight loss efforts. On the other hand, those with higher self-esteem may be more confident in their ability to stick to a healthy diet and exercise routine.

It's important to remember that weight loss is not just about the numbers on the scale. It's also about making positive changes to your overall health and well-being. This can involve adopting healthy habits such as eating a balanced diet, getting regular physical activity, and managing stress.

Setting realistic goals and establishing a plan for achieving them can also be helpful. This might include setting a goal for how much weight you want to lose, as well as smaller goals along the way. Having a plan in place can help you stay on track and make progress towards your overall goal.

It's important to be patient and kind to yourself during the weight loss process. Weight loss can be a challenging journey, and there may be setbacks and setbacks along the way. It's important to remember that it's okay to have setbacks and that it's normal to have ups and downs. What's important is to keep moving forward and to stay motivated and focused on your goals.

If you're struggling with weight loss, it can be helpful to seek support from a professional, such as a therapist or registered dietitian. They can help you identify and address any underlying emotional or psychological issues that may be contributing to your challenges and provide you with tools and strategies to help you achieve your weight loss goals.

In conclusion, understanding the psychology of weight loss can be a valuable tool in your journey towards a healthy weight. By focusing on motivation, self-regulation, mindfulness, and support, you can develop the skills and strategies needed to successfully lose weight and maintain a healthy lifestyle.

Weight loss is a complex topic that goes beyond calories and exercise. It involves deep-seated emotions, beliefs, and societal pressures that influence our behaviors and decisions. In this chapter, we will explore the psychological factors that play a critical role in weight loss and discuss why understanding these elements is key to achieving a sustainable, no-diet approach to health.

Important Key points:

The Influence of Diet Culture: Diet culture has shaped our understanding of weight loss, often promoting quick fixes, restrictive diets, and unrealistic body standards. This culture creates a cycle of guilt and shame around food, leading many people to adopt unhealthy patterns in their pursuit of weight loss. By focusing solely on the physical aspects of losing weight, diet culture overlooks the psychological complexities that can drive unhealthy behaviors.

The Role of Emotions in Eating: Emotions play a significant role in our eating habits. Stress, anxiety, sadness, or even boredom can lead to emotional eating, where food is used to cope with negative feelings. This emotional reliance on food can hinder weight loss efforts and perpetuate a cycle of overeating, followed by guilt and restrictive dieting. To break this cycle, it's important to understand the emotional triggers behind eating patterns and develop healthier coping mechanisms.

Beliefs and Self-Perception: Our beliefs about ourselves and our bodies can greatly impact our ability to lose weight. Negative self-perception, body shaming, and low self-esteem often lead to destructive behaviors like binge eating or extreme dieting. Understanding these beliefs and working to change them is crucial for a successful weight loss journey. A positive self-image and acceptance can help break free from the negative thought patterns that hold us back.

The Impact of Social Support: Social support can significantly influence weight loss success. Surrounding yourself with positive influences—friends, family, or support groups—can provide encouragement and accountability. This support system can help you stay motivated, celebrate achievements, and navigate setbacks. It also helps combat the isolation that often accompanies traditional dieting.

Developing a Growth Mindset: A growth mindset is essential for successful weight loss. This mindset embraces challenges, learns from failures, and views effort as the path to mastery. Instead of fixating on setbacks or mistakes, those with a growth mindset see them as opportunities for growth and improvement. Adopting this mindset can transform the weight loss journey from a battle with oneself into a journey of self-discovery and empowerment.

The Importance of Mindful Eating: Mindful eating is a practice that can significantly improve the psychological relationship with food. By being present during meals, savoring each bite, and listening to hunger and fullness cues, you can develop a healthier approach to eating. This practice helps you enjoy food without guilt and reduces the likelihood of overeating or binge eating.

Understanding the psychology of weight loss is a critical step in creating a sustainable, no-diet approach to health. By recognizing the influence of diet culture, managing emotional eating, changing negative beliefs, and fostering a growth mindset, you can lay the foundation for a successful weight loss journey. In the following chapters, we will explore how to apply these psychological principles to create a balanced, enjoyable, and long-lasting approach to health and well-being.

CHAPTER TWO

The Truth About Dieting and Weight Loss

One of the biggest myths about weight loss is that it's as simple as calories in, calories out. But the truth is, losing weight and maintaining a healthy weight is much more complex than that.

In this chapter, we'll explore the truth about dieting and weight loss and debunk some of the most common myths and misconceptions. You'll learn about the role that genetics, metabolism, and other factors play in weight management, and how to find a healthy approach to weight loss that works for you.

One of the biggest mistakes people make when trying to lose weight is falling for fad diets and quick fixes. These approaches may promise rapid weight loss, but they are often unsustainable and can even be dangerous. In the long run, they can lead to weight cycling, also known as yo-yo dieting, which can have negative effects on your health and well-being.

Instead of following a restrictive, one-size-fits-all diet plan, it's important to find a healthy, sustainable approach to weight loss that works for you. This might involve making small, gradual changes to your eating and exercise habits, or seeking the support of a registered dietitian or other healthcare professional.

By understanding the truth about dieting and weight loss, you'll be better equipped to navigate the confusing world of weight loss advice and find a healthy approach that works for you.

Another common myth about weight loss is that all calories are created equal. This couldn't be further from the truth. The quality of the calories you consume can have a big impact on your weight and overall health.

For example, calories from nutrient-dense, whole foods like fruits, vegetables, whole grains, and lean proteins are more likely to satisfy your hunger and provide your body with the nutrients it needs to function properly. On the other hand, calories from processed, high-fat, and high-sugar foods are less likely to satisfy your hunger and may contribute to weight gain.

This doesn't mean you have to eliminate all of your favorite foods in order to lose weight. In fact, one of the key principles of "The No-Diet Diet" is learning to enjoy the foods you love in moderation. But it does mean paying attention to the quality of the calories you consume and finding a balance that works for you.

Weight management is a complex process that is influenced by a variety of factors, including genetics, metabolism, and lifestyle.

Genetics can play a role in weight management by influencing factors such as appetite, metabolism, and the distribution of fat in the body. Some people may have a genetic predisposition to gain weight more easily or to have a slower metabolism, which can make it more challenging to maintain a healthy weight. However, genetics is only one piece of the puzzle, and lifestyle factors, such as diet and exercise, can also significantly impact weight management.

Metabolism is the process by which the body converts food into energy. It can also influence weight management, as a faster metabolism may help the body burn calories more efficiently, while a slower metabolism may make it more difficult to lose weight. However, metabolism can be influenced by various factors, such as age, hormone levels, and physical activity, so it is not the only determinant of weight.

Other factors that can affect weight management include lifestyle factors such as sleep patterns, stress levels, and the quality of the foods you eat. It's important to consider all of these factors when trying to lose weight and maintain a healthy weight.

In order to find a healthy approach to weight loss that works for you, it is important to focus on making sustainable lifestyle changes rather than trying fad diets or quick fixes. This may include incorporating regular physical activity into your routine, eating a balanced diet that is rich in fruits, vegetables, and lean proteins, and getting enough sleep. It can also be helpful to work with a healthcare professional or a registered dietitian to develop a plan that is tailored to your individual needs and goals.

Ultimately, the key to successful weight management is finding a healthy and sustainable approach that works for you, rather than relying on quick fixes or drastic measures. By making healthy lifestyle choices and seeking support when needed, you can improve your overall health and well-being, and achieve and maintain a healthy weight.

One key component of a healthy approach to weight loss is incorporating regular physical activity into your routine. This can help to boost metabolism, burn calories, and improve overall health. Aim for at least 150 minutes of moderate intensity activity or 75 minutes of vigorous intensity activity each week, as recommended by the Centers for Disease Control and Prevention (CDC). This can include activities such as walking, running, cycling, swimming, or participating in a sport or fitness class.

In addition to regular physical activity, a healthy diet is also important for weight loss. This can include eating a variety of nutrient-dense foods, such as fruits, vegetables, lean proteins, whole grains, and healthy fats. It can also be helpful to limit your intake of added sugars, processed foods, and unhealthy fats. Paying attention to portion sizes and eating mindfully can also be helpful in managing your weight.

Other lifestyle factors that can impact weight loss include getting enough sleep, managing stress, and staying hydrated. Aim for 7-9 hours of sleep per night, practice stress-reducing techniques such as meditation or yoga, and drink plenty of water throughout the day to support healthy weight management.

It can also be helpful to seek support from a healthcare professional or a registered dietitian when trying to lose weight. They can provide guidance and support to help you develop a plan that is tailored to your individual needs and goals.

Overall, the key to a healthy approach to weight loss is making sustainable lifestyle changes that are sustainable and support overall health and well-being. By focusing on a balanced diet, regular physical activity, and other healthy habits, you can successfully lose weight and improve your overall health.

In addition to regular physical activity and a healthy diet, there are several other strategies that can help you achieve a healthy weight and maintain it over time. Here are a few tips to consider:

Eat mindfully: Pay attention to what you eat, and try to avoid distractions such as screens or multitasking while eating. This can help you to be more aware of your food choices and portion sizes, and to better enjoy your meals.

Choose nutrient-dense foods: Instead of focusing on calories alone, aim to include a variety of nutrient-dense foods in your diet. These are foods that are high in nutrients relative to their calorie content, such as fruits, vegetables, lean proteins, and whole grains.

Plan ahead: Planning your meals and snacks in advance can help you to make healthier choices and to avoid last-minute, unhealthy options. You can also try prepping meals in advance or packing healthy snacks to take with you when you're on the go.

Get support: It can be helpful to enlist the support of friends, family, or a healthcare professional or registered dietitian when trying to lose weight. They can provide encouragement, accountability, and guidance to help you stay on track.

Be patient and consistent: Weight loss can take time, and it's important to be patient and consistent in your efforts. Don't get discouraged if you don't see immediate results, and remember that small, sustainable changes are more likely to be successful in the long term.

Remember that everyone is different, and what works for one person may not work for another. It's important to find a healthy approach to weight loss that works for you and meets your individual needs and goals. With patience, consistency, and the right support, you can achieve a healthy weight and maintain it over time.

Dieting has become synonymous with weight loss, yet its true impact is often misunderstood. In this chapter, we will uncover the reality of dieting and explore why conventional approaches to weight loss can be harmful in the long run. We will examine the myths and facts about dieting and offer insights into a more sustainable way to achieve and maintain a healthy weight.

Important Key points:

The Dieting Paradox

One of the most surprising truths about dieting is the "dieting paradox": many people who diet end up gaining weight over time. This paradox occurs because restrictive diets often trigger a cycle of deprivation, overeating, and guilt, leading to a yo-yo effect where weight fluctuates rather than stabilizes. The more someone diets, the more likely they are to experience this cycle, making long-term weight loss challenging.

The Myths of Quick Fixes

Diet culture promotes the idea that quick-fix diets can produce rapid weight loss. However, these approaches often rely on extreme calorie restriction, elimination of food groups, or unsustainable practices that can harm physical and mental health. The truth is that weight loss requires time, patience, and a balanced approach. Quick-fix diets rarely lead to permanent results and can cause more harm than good.

The Impact of Restrictive Diets

Restrictive diets can have a significant impact on the body and mind. Physically, they can lead to nutrient deficiencies, decreased energy, and metabolic slowdown. Mentally, they can foster unhealthy relationships with food, cause emotional distress, and lead to disordered eating patterns. The more restrictive a diet, the more likely it is to cause stress and ultimately fail.

The Role of Metabolism

Metabolism plays a crucial role in weight loss, but many diets neglect its importance. Extreme calorie restriction can slow metabolism, making it harder to lose weight and easier to gain it back. Diets that focus on maintaining a healthy metabolism through balanced nutrition, regular exercise, and adequate rest are more likely to yield sustainable results.

Sustainable Approaches to Weight Loss

The truth about dieting is that sustainable weight loss requires a holistic approach. This approach focuses on balanced nutrition, regular physical activity, and a healthy mindset. Instead of drastic changes, sustainable approaches encourage gradual shifts in habits that can be maintained over time. This includes eating a variety of foods, staying active, managing stress, and fostering a positive relationship with food.

The Importance of Individualization

No single diet works for everyone. Each person's body, metabolism, and lifestyle are unique, and so are their dietary needs. The truth about dieting is that individualization is key. Sustainable weight loss involves understanding your body's needs, listening to your hunger and fullness cues, and finding an approach that aligns with your preferences and goals.

The truth about dieting and weight loss is that there are no shortcuts or one-size-fits-all solutions. Restrictive diets and quick-fix approaches often lead to failure and frustration. By embracing a sustainable, individualized approach, you can create lasting change that promotes health and well-being. In the following chapters, we will explore practical strategies to help you develop a no-diet approach to weight loss that focuses on balance, mindfulness, and overall health.

CHAPTER THREE

Finding Your Own Path to Weight Loss Success

In this chapter, we'll discuss the importance of individuality and the role that personal preferences, goals, and lifestyle play in weight loss. You'll learn how to assess your own needs and find a healthy, sustainable approach to weight loss that works for you.

One key to finding your own path to weight loss success is to ditch the strict rules and unrealistic goals. Instead of trying to follow a rigid diet plan or exercise regimen, focus on finding a healthy balance that works for you. This might involve making small, gradual changes to your eating and exercise habits, or seeking the support of a registered dietitian or other healthcare professional.

Another important aspect of finding your own path is to focus on progress, not perfection. It's important to remember that progress is not always linear and it's okay to have setbacks along the way. By embracing a journey mentality and practicing self-compassion, you'll be more likely to persevere and ultimately achieve your weight loss goals.

Losing weight can be a challenging and daunting task, but it is also an incredibly rewarding and beneficial journey for both your physical and mental health. While there are many different approaches to weight loss, the most successful weight loss journey is one that is tailored to your unique needs, preferences, and lifestyle. Here are some tips to help you find your own path to weight loss success:

Set specific and achievable goals: It's important to set specific and achievable weight loss goals to help keep you motivated and on track. Consider consulting with a healthcare professional to determine a healthy and realistic target weight for your height, age, and body composition.

Find a weight loss plan that works for you: There are many different approaches to weight loss, such as low-carb diets, low-fat diets, and meal replacement programs. It's important to find a plan that fits your lifestyle and preferences and that you can realistically stick to over the long term.

Incorporate physical activity: Regular physical activity is an essential component of any successful weight loss journey. Aim for at least 150 minutes of moderate-intensity activity, such as brisk walking or cycling, per week. You can also incorporate strength training, such as lifting weights or using resistance bands, to help build muscle and boost metabolism.

Make healthy lifestyle choices: In addition to following a healthy diet and being physically active, other lifestyle factors can also contribute to successful weight loss. These include getting enough sleep, managing stress, and staying hydrated.

Seek support: Losing weight can be a challenging and emotional process, and it can be helpful to have the support of friends, family, or a support group. Consider joining a weight loss program or seeking the guidance of a healthcare professional or a licensed therapist.

Keep a food diary: Tracking your food intake can be a useful tool for identifying areas where you may be able to make healthier choices. Consider keeping a food diary or using a food tracking app to help you become more aware of your eating habits. For example, you may realize that you tend to snack on unhealthy foods when you're feeling stressed or bored. By identifying these triggers, you can find healthier ways to cope with emotions or find alternative activities to do instead of snacking.

Experiment with different types of exercise: Not everyone enjoys the same types of physical activity, so it's important to find activities that you enjoy and that keep you motivated. Consider trying a variety of exercises, such as dancing, swimming, or hiking, to see what works best for you. For example, you may discover that you love the feeling of accomplishment you get from lifting weights, or that you enjoy the meditative aspect of yoga.

Don't be afraid to seek professional help: If you're struggling to lose weight on your own, it can be helpful to seek the guidance of a healthcare professional or a licensed therapist. A healthcare professional can help you assess your current eating and exercise habits and provide personalized recommendations for reaching your weight loss goals. A therapist can also help you address any underlying emotional or psychological issues that may be contributing to your weight gain.

Make healthy eating a priority: Instead of depriving yourself of the foods you love, focus on incorporating more whole, nutrient-dense foods into your diet. Aim for a balanced intake of fruits, vegetables, lean proteins, and whole grains. For example, instead of ordering a fast food burger and fries for lunch, try packing a turkey and avocado sandwich on whole grain bread with a side of fruit.

Don't compare yourself to others: It's important to remember that everyone's weight loss journey is unique and that progress may not always be linear. Instead of comparing yourself to others, focus on your own progress and celebrate your own accomplishments.

Remember, losing weight is a journey and it's important to be patient and kind to yourself. It's okay to have setbacks or slip-ups – it's how you handle them that matters. Stay positive and focus on the progress you've made, and you will eventually reach your weight loss goals.

Important Key points:

Identifying Your Goals

The first step in finding your own path to weight loss success is identifying your goals. These goals should reflect what you truly want to achieve, whether it's improved health, increased energy, or a specific fitness milestone. The key is to make them specific, measurable, achievable, relevant, and time-bound (SMART). This way, you can track your progress and stay motivated throughout your journey.

Embracing Flexibility and Individuality

A successful weight loss journey requires flexibility and an understanding of your unique needs. Recognize that what works for one person may not work for another. Embrace the idea that your journey can evolve and adapt to your changing circumstances. This flexibility can help you avoid the frustration that comes from rigid, one-size-fits-all diets.

Building Healthy Habits

Creating healthy habits is crucial for sustainable weight loss. Instead of focusing on dramatic changes, concentrate on small, manageable adjustments that can be maintained over time. This might involve incorporating more vegetables into your meals, finding enjoyable forms of exercise, or setting aside time for mindfulness and relaxation. The goal is to create a lifestyle that supports your health and well-being.

Finding Support and Accountability

Having a support system is vital to weight loss success. This support can come from friends, family, or a community of like-minded individuals. Look for people who encourage you, share your goals, and hold you accountable. Consider joining a fitness class, an online group, or working with a coach to stay on track and motivated.

Practicing Mindful Eating

Mindful eating is an essential component of finding your path to weight loss success. It involves paying attention to your hunger and fullness cues, savoring your meals, and eating without distractions. By practicing mindful eating, you can build a healthier relationship with food and reduce the likelihood of overeating or emotional eating.

Overcoming Setbacks

Setbacks are a natural part of any weight loss journey. The key is to view them as learning opportunities rather than failures. When you encounter a setback, reflect on what happened, identify any triggers or patterns, and develop a plan to address them in the future. This approach helps you stay resilient and focused on your long-term goals.

Finding your own path to weight loss success is about embracing your individuality, building sustainable habits, and creating a supportive environment. By setting realistic goals, practicing mindful eating, and staying flexible, you can develop a personalized approach that leads to lasting results. In the following chapters, we'll delve deeper into specific strategies and techniques to help you continue on your unique journey toward a healthier, happier you.

CHAPTER FOUR

The Importance of Balance and Moderation

One of the key principles of "The No-Diet Diet" is the importance of balance and moderation. In this chapter, we'll discuss why these concepts are so crucial to weight loss and overall health, and provide practical tips and strategies for incorporating them into your life.

Maintaining balance and moderation in regards to weight loss is important for a number of reasons. First, when it comes to dieting, it's important to find a balance between calorie restriction and nutrient-dense foods. It's possible to lose weight through extreme calorie restriction, but this often leads to feelings of deprivation and can be difficult to sustain over the long term. It's generally more effective to aim for a moderate calorie deficit while still ensuring that you're getting all the nutrients your body needs.

In addition to balanced eating, it's also important to find balance in your overall lifestyle. This includes balancing physical activity with rest, work with leisure, and finding ways to manage stress. All of these factors can impact weight loss, and it's important to find a balance that works for you.

Moderation is also key when it comes to weight loss. Extreme or restrictive diets are often not sustainable over the long term, and it's important to find a way of eating that you can stick to for the long haul. This often means allowing yourself to indulge in your favorite foods in moderation, rather than completely cutting them out of your diet.

Another reason why balance and moderation are important in weight loss is that they can help to prevent the yo-yo effect, where a person loses weight only to gain it back and then some. This can be frustrating and demoralizing, and can lead to a negative relationship with food and one's body.

Maintaining balance and moderation can help to prevent the yo-yo effect by ensuring that weight loss is gradual and sustainable. It's generally recommended to aim for a weight loss of 1-2 pounds per week, as this is a realistic and achievable goal that can be maintained over the long term.

In addition to helping with weight loss, balance and moderation can also have a number of other benefits for overall health and well-being. Eating a balanced diet can help to ensure that you're getting all the nutrients your body needs to function properly, and can also help to reduce the risk of certain health conditions such as heart disease and type 2 diabetes.

Finding balance in your overall lifestyle can also help to reduce stress and improve overall well-being. Engaging in physical activity, getting enough sleep, and finding ways to manage stress can all contribute to better mental and physical health.

Overall, balance and moderation are important in weight loss because they help you to create a healthy, sustainable lifestyle that you can maintain over the long term. This can help you to not only lose weight, but also to maintain your weight loss and improve your overall health and well-being.

Important Key points:

Understanding Balance and Moderation

Balance and moderation involve finding harmony in your diet and lifestyle. This means including a variety of foods, engaging in regular physical activity, and allowing yourself to enjoy life without excessive restrictions. It's about creating a sustainable approach that prioritizes health and well-being over drastic measures or extreme dieting.

The Risks of Extreme Dieting

Extreme dieting, such as very low-calorie diets, food group elimination, or intense exercise regimens, can lead to adverse health effects. These risks include nutrient deficiencies, muscle loss, fatigue, and even psychological stress. Furthermore, extreme approaches are often unsustainable, leading to yo-yo dieting and feelings of failure. Understanding the risks can help you embrace a more balanced and moderate path.

Achieving Nutritional Balance

Nutritional balance is a core aspect of moderation. This involves consuming a variety of food groups, including carbohydrates, proteins, fats, vitamins, and minerals. A balanced diet ensures that your body receives all the necessary nutrients to function optimally. Instead of categorizing foods as "good" or "bad," focus on variety and quality. This approach promotes a healthier relationship with food and reduces the temptation to binge or restrict.

Incorporating Treats and Indulgences

Moderation includes allowing yourself to enjoy treats and indulgences without guilt. Completely depriving yourself of favorite foods often leads to cravings and eventual overeating. Instead, practice mindful indulgence—savoring your favorite dessert, snack, or meal occasionally. This approach helps you maintain a balanced mindset, reduces the allure of "forbidden" foods, and fosters a more sustainable relationship with eating.

Balancing Physical Activity

Physical activity is essential for a healthy lifestyle, but balance is key. Overtraining or excessive exercise can lead to burnout, injury, and decreased motivation. Instead, aim for a varied exercise routine that includes cardio, strength training, and flexibility exercises. Find activities you enjoy, whether it's dancing, hiking, yoga, or sports. This balanced approach to exercise supports weight loss while enhancing overall health and well-being.

Mindset and Moderation

Your mindset plays a critical role in maintaining balance and moderation. A rigid, all-or-nothing mindset can lead to unrealistic expectations and disappointment. Instead, adopt a flexible mindset that allows for occasional deviations from your plan without derailing your progress. This mindset fosters resilience and keeps you on track even when faced with challenges or setbacks.

CHAPTER FIVE

How to listen to your body's hunger and fullness cues

It's important to listen to your body's hunger and fullness cues when trying to lose weight or maintain a healthy diet. Doing so can help you maintain a healthy weight and make sure you're getting the nutrients you need. Here are some tips for listening to your body's hunger and fullness cues:

Eat when you're hungry: Pay attention to your body's hunger cues and eat when you feel hungry. It's okay to feel hungry between meals – this is your body's way of telling you it needs fuel.

Stop eating when you're full: Pay attention to your body's fullness cues and stop eating when you feel satisfied, rather than stuffed. It can take your brain a while to catch up with your stomach, so try to stop eating before you feel overly full.

Don't skip meals: Skipping meals can lead to overeating later on, as your body tries to make up for the missed calories. Try to eat regular, balanced meals to keep your hunger in check.

Eat slowly: It takes time for your brain to register that your stomach is full, so try eating slowly to give it time to catch up. This can help you stop eating when you're full, rather than continuing to eat until you feel stuffed.

Drink water: Staying hydrated can help you feel full and satisfied, so make sure to drink plenty of water throughout the day.

Distinguish emotional hunger from physical hunger: Sometimes people eat not because they are physically hungry but because of emotional reasons like stress, boredom, or anxiety. It's important to recognize the difference between emotional hunger and physical hunger, so you can address the underlying emotional issue rather than using food as a coping mechanism. When you feel an urge to eat, take a moment to ask yourself if you're truly hungry or if there's something else going on.

Keep a food diary: Keeping a food diary can help you track your eating habits and identify patterns. You can use it to record what you eat, when you eat, and how hungry or full you feel at different times of the day. This can help you see where you're going wrong and make adjustments to your eating habits.

Learn to cook: Cooking your own meals at home can be a great way to ensure that you're eating nutritious, well-balanced meals. It also gives you more control over the ingredients and portion sizes, which can be helpful if you're trying to lose weight.

Be mindful: Mindfulness is the practice of paying attention to the present moment without judgment. When you eat, try to focus on the food and your body's signals, rather than multitasking or getting lost in your thoughts. This can help you enjoy your food more and make better decisions about how much to eat.

Seek professional help: If you're struggling to lose weight or maintain a healthy diet, consider seeking professional help. A registered dietitian or a therapist can provide guidance and support to help you reach your goals.

Let's take an example of Sarah, who is trying to lose weight and improve her overall health.

Sarah starts by paying attention to her body's hunger and fullness cues, she makes sure to eat when she's hungry and stop eating when she's full. She also starts to notice that sometimes she reaches for food when she's not truly hungry, but when she's feeling bored or stressed. To help address this, she starts practicing mindfulness during meals and takes a moment to ask herself if she's truly hungry before eating.

Sarah also starts keeping a food diary, recording what she eats, when she eats, and how hungry or full she feels at different times of the day. By reviewing her food diary, she notices that she tends to overeat at night, especially when she's watching TV. She makes the decision to keep her evening meals small, and find alternative ways to relax and unwind in the evenings.

Sarah also learns to cook, this allows her to have better control over her meals, she starts to make healthy and balanced meals at home, this also helps her save money and time.

Sarah also drinks water and tries to stay hydrated as much as possible. Drinking water helps her to stay full and satisfied, and she finds that it helps her to make better decisions about when to stop eating.

Sarah also finds that she would benefit from seeing a registered dietitian for additional guidance and support. With the help of a professional, Sarah is able to make a personalized meal plan that takes into account her individual needs and goals.

Sarah is also aware that progress takes time and effort, and she's prepared to make mistakes along the way. She's kind and compassionate with herself, and she understands that it's all part of the process. With patience and perseverance, Sarah eventually reaches her weight loss and health goals.

Another important aspect of weight loss and dieting is exercise. Regular physical activity can help boost weight loss and improve overall health. Sarah starts incorporating regular exercise into her routine, aiming for at least 30 minutes of moderate-intensity activity most days of the week. She finds that she enjoys going for a brisk walk or jog in the morning, and she joins a local gym to try out different exercise classes like yoga or strength training.

Sarah also starts paying more attention to the quality of the food she eats, focusing on nutrient-dense foods such as fruits, vegetables, lean proteins, and whole grains. She reduces her intake of processed foods and added sugars, which not only help with weight loss but also with her overall health.

Sarah also starts to be more mindful of her portion sizes, and learns how to estimate appropriate serving sizes. She uses measuring cups and a food scale to help her get a better sense of the right portions. She also becomes more aware of the calorie content of the foods she eats and starts to make healthier choices when eating out.

Another way Sarah helps herself to stick to her diet and weight loss journey is by creating accountability for herself. She tells her friends and family about her goals, and finds a support group either in person or online, where she can connect with people who are also working on losing weight and getting healthy. This helps her to stay motivated and on track, and she finds that having people to talk to who understand what she's going through is incredibly helpful.

In summary, listening to your body's hunger and fullness cues, keeping track of your food intake, eating nutrient-dense foods, being mindful of portion sizes, incorporating regular exercise, and seeking professional help are key steps that Sarah takes to help her reach her weight loss and health goals. It's also important to remember that progress takes time, and that it's okay to make mistakes along the way. With patience, perseverance and the right tools, anyone can achieve their weight loss and health goals.

By paying attention to your body's hunger and fullness cues, you can make sure you're eating enough to fuel your body without overdoing it. This can help you maintain a healthy weight and overall sense of well-being.

Many people have lost touch with their natural hunger and fullness cues due to factors like stress, busy schedules, emotional eating, or years of following restrictive diets. Reconnecting with these cues is a critical step in creating a balanced and mindful approach to eating.

Understanding your body's signals starts with differentiating between physical hunger and emotional hunger. Physical hunger is your body's way of signaling that it needs nourishment. It can manifest as stomach growling, light-headedness, or a drop in energy. Emotional hunger, on the other hand, is often triggered by stress, boredom, or other emotional factors, leading to cravings for comfort foods or mindless eating. Learning to recognize these differences is key to making more informed eating choices.

To tune into your hunger cues, begin by observing your body's signals throughout the day. When you feel hungry, ask yourself if it's been a while since you last ate, or if there might be an emotional trigger causing the sensation. If you're physically hungry, opt for a balanced meal or snack. If it's emotional hunger, consider other ways to address your emotions, like taking a walk, talking to a friend, or practicing relaxation techniques.

Similarly, understanding your body's fullness cues is crucial. Fullness signals can include a feeling of satiety, reduced interest in food, or a comfortable sensation in your stomach. To avoid overeating, practice eating slowly and paying attention to these cues during meals. Taking small breaks to assess your level of fullness can help you recognize when you've had enough to eat.

Practicing mindful eating can greatly enhance your ability to listen to hunger and fullness cues. Mindful eating involves being present during meals, savoring each bite, and minimizing distractions. By focusing on the flavors, textures, and smells of your food, you create a deeper connection with what you're eating. This approach helps you enjoy your meals more and reduces the likelihood of overeating or mindless snacking.

Another helpful technique is to use a hunger and fullness scale. This scale typically ranges from 1 to 10, with 1 being extremely hungry and 10 being uncomfortably full. Aim to eat when you're moderately hungry, around a 3 or 4, and stop when you're comfortably full, around a 7 or 8. Using this scale can provide a practical way to gauge your body's cues and make adjustments as needed.

Listening to your body's hunger and fullness cues requires practice and patience. It might take time to rebuild this awareness, especially if you've been accustomed to rigid dieting or emotional eating. Be patient with yourself, and remember that the goal is to create a healthier, more intuitive relationship with food.

By learning to listen to your body, you can make more mindful choices, improve your eating habits, and ultimately achieve a more balanced and sustainable approach to weight loss. In the following chapters, we'll explore additional strategies and techniques to support your journey towards a healthier and happier lifestyle.

CHAPTER SIX

Making healthy eating choices without feeling deprived

Eating healthy is a crucial part of any weight loss journey, but it can be easy to feel deprived when making changes to your diet. However, there are ways to make healthy eating choices without feeling deprived.

One of the key strategies for avoiding feelings of deprivation is to focus on the benefits of healthy eating rather than on the foods that you can no longer eat. For example, instead of thinking about all the junk food that you can't have, focus on the fact that by eating more fruits and vegetables, you'll be getting essential vitamins and minerals that will help you feel better and have more energy.

Another strategy is to find healthy substitutes for your favorite foods. For example, if you love pizza, try making a cauliflower crust pizza. If you're craving chocolate, try a piece of dark chocolate or a small serving of chocolate-covered berries. There are many healthy substitutions that can help curb cravings and keep you feeling satisfied.

It's also important to remember that healthy eating is about balance and moderation. Depriving yourself of all the foods you love is not sustainable, and will only lead to feelings of deprivation and cravings. Instead, allow yourself to indulge in small amounts of your favorite foods every once in a while. This can help you feel like you're still enjoying the foods you love while still making progress towards your weight loss goals.

It's also helpful to pay attention to your body's natural hunger and fullness cues. Instead of eating because you're bored or stressed, focus on eating when you're actually hungry and stop eating when you're full. This can help you to be more mindful of your eating habits and to be more in tune with your body's natural hunger and fullness signals.

Additionally, Engage in regular physical activity, which can help boost your mood, reduce stress, and burn calories. Whether you enjoy going for a walk, running, swimming, or hitting the gym, finding an exercise that you enjoy can help you stay motivated and on track with your weight loss goals.

Another important aspect of making healthy eating choices without feeling deprived is to plan ahead. This can help you to stay on track with your weight loss goals and avoid making poor food choices when you're feeling rushed or stressed.

For example, you can plan your meals for the week in advance and make sure that you have all the ingredients you need on hand. You can also pack healthy snacks, like fruits or vegetables, to take with you when you're on the go. This can help you to avoid reaching for unhealthy foods when you're feeling hungry and don't have anything healthy to eat.

It's also a good idea to take the time to learn more about nutrition and healthy eating. The more you understand about the foods you're eating and their nutritional value, the more equipped you'll be to make healthy choices. You can look up recipes and articles, watch cooking shows and lectures on the topic, or even consider consulting a dietician or nutritionist who can provide personalized recommendations.

Another way to make healthy eating choices without feeling deprived is to focus on the pleasure and social aspects of eating. Eating is not only about fuel but also pleasure, bonding, culture and traditions. Try to cook and eat with friends or family and make it a social activity. You can even try new cuisines and cooking styles, experiment with spices, and find new healthy dishes that you enjoy. Make healthy eating an enjoyable experience rather than a punishment.

Finally, it's important to be patient and kind to yourself. Making changes to your diet and losing weight can be challenging, and it's important to remember that progress takes time. Be patient with yourself and don't beat yourself up if you slip up or make a mistake. Instead, focus on the progress that you've made and continue to make healthier choices moving forward.

It's possible to make healthy eating choices and lose weight without feeling deprived by focusing on the benefits of healthy eating, finding healthy substitutes, and allowing yourself to indulge in small amounts, paying attention to your body's natural hunger and fullness cues and being active. Making healthy eating choices and losing weight without feeling deprived requires a holistic approach. It's not only about the food itself, but also about our mindset, emotions, habits and social context. It's important to find healthy substitutes, plan ahead, educate yourself, make eating social, and most importantly, be patient and kind to yourself. Remember, making progress towards your weight loss goals is more important than perfection, it is a journey and progress is what counts, not perfection.

Sarah is a 35-year-old woman who has been struggling to lose weight for several years. She wants to make healthy eating choices without feeling deprived, but she's not sure how to get started. Here's an example of how Sarah can approach her weight loss journey in a sustainable way:

First, Sarah should start by setting realistic goals for herself. Instead of trying to lose a significant amount of weight quickly, she should aim to lose 1-2 pounds per week. This will help her to focus on progress instead of perfection and avoid feelings of deprivation.

Next, Sarah should focus on the benefits of healthy eating. She could make a list of all the benefits she hopes to achieve, such as having more energy, reducing her risk of chronic diseases, or fitting into her favorite clothes. Keeping this list in a place where she can see it every day will remind her of why she's making these changes and help her to stay motivated.

Sarah should then find healthy substitutes for her favorite foods. For example, instead of eating a bag of potato chips as a snack, she could try making her own baked sweet potato chips or snacking on veggies with a hummus dip. This will help her to curb her cravings without feeling deprived.

Sarah should also make sure to allow herself to indulge in small amounts of her favorite foods every once in a while. For example, she could have a small serving of ice cream on the weekends or a piece of cake on her birthday. This will help her to feel like she's still enjoying the foods she loves while still making progress towards her weight loss goals.

Sarah should also pay attention to her body's natural hunger and fullness cues. Instead of eating when she's not hungry, she should eat when she's actually hungry and stop eating when she's full. This will help her to be more mindful of her eating habits and to be more in tune with her body's natural hunger and fullness signals.

Finally, Sarah should make sure to engage in regular physical activity. This can help boost her mood, reduce stress, and burn calories. She could try different activities and find what she enjoys like going for a walk, running, swimming, or hitting the gym. Sarah can make healthy eating choices and lose weight without feeling deprived by setting realistic goals, focusing on the benefits of healthy eating, finding healthy substitutes, allowing herself to indulge in small amounts, paying attention to her body's natural hunger and fullness cues, and engaging in regular physical activity. With this approach, Sarah can lose weight in a sustainable way and feel good about the progress she makes.

Another strategy for Sarah to make healthy eating choices without feeling deprived is to plan ahead. She can plan her meals for the week in advance, making a grocery list of all the ingredients she needs, so she can always have healthy food options at home. By planning ahead, Sarah will be more prepared for any situation and will avoid impulse buying or reaching for unhealthy options when she's feeling rushed or stressed.

Sarah can also take the time to educate herself about nutrition and healthy eating. She can research different foods, their nutritional value and how to prepare them. She can try new recipes and explore different cuisines, this will not only make her meals more interesting and diverse, but also will give her the chance to find new healthy dishes that she likes.

Another important aspect to focus on is the pleasure and social aspects of eating. Eating is not only about fueling our bodies, but also it is an opportunity to bond with others and enjoy the company of friends and family.

Sarah could try to cook and eat together with friends or family. She can even take cooking classes or join a cooking group where she can learn new skills, share experiences and make new friends who have similar interests.

Additionally, it's important to be patient and kind to herself, weight loss journeys can be challenging and progress might not always be linear. It's important for Sarah to remember that progress takes time and she may slip up or make mistakes, but that doesn't mean she should give up. Instead, Sarah should focus on what she has accomplished, be proud of her progress, and continue to make healthier choices moving forward.

In conclusion, Making healthy eating choices without feeling deprived is a journey, and it's important to take a holistic approach that covers both physical and emotional aspects. Sarah can set realistic goals, focus on the benefits of healthy eating, find healthy substitutes, allow herself to indulge in small amounts, pay attention to her body's natural hunger and fullness cues, engage in regular physical activity, plan ahead, educate herself, make eating a social and enjoyable experience and most importantly, be patient and kind to herself.

Eating healthily doesn't have to mean feeling deprived. It's possible to create a balanced diet that satisfies your nutritional needs without sacrificing enjoyment. In this chapter, we'll discuss how to make healthy eating choices while still enjoying food, explore ways to cultivate a positive relationship with meals, and address common pitfalls that lead to feelings of deprivation.

One of the key aspects of making healthy eating choices without feeling deprived is adopting a flexible and balanced approach to nutrition. Rather than categorizing foods as "good" or "bad," embrace the concept of variety and moderation. By including a wide range of foods in your diet, you avoid the rigidity of restrictive eating plans, which often lead to cravings and a sense of deprivation.

A practical way to make healthier choices is to focus on adding nutrient-rich foods to your meals, rather than eliminating entire food groups. Incorporate more vegetables, fruits, whole grains, and lean proteins into your diet. This way, you can increase the nutritional value of your meals without restricting yourself from enjoying your favorite foods.

Another important strategy is to create meals that are both nutritious and enjoyable. Healthy eating doesn't mean eating bland or boring food. Experiment with herbs, spices, and different cooking techniques to make your meals flavorful and interesting. Try new recipes and cuisines to keep things exciting, and don't be afraid to indulge in occasional treats. This approach helps you maintain a positive relationship with food and reduces the temptation to binge on "forbidden" items.

Mindful eating can also play a significant role in reducing feelings of deprivation. By eating mindfully, you focus on the present moment and savor the flavors and textures of your food. This practice encourages you to eat more slowly, allowing you to better recognize hunger and fullness cues. It can also enhance your enjoyment of meals, leading to greater satisfaction with smaller portions.

Social factors can influence your perception of healthy eating. If your social circle often engages in unhealthy eating habits, it can be challenging to maintain your own goals. To combat this, surround yourself with supportive people who share your values around health and nutrition. Engage in activities and events that promote healthy eating, and don't be afraid to suggest alternative venues or meals when dining out with friends or family.

To avoid deprivation, it's crucial to allow yourself the flexibility to enjoy occasional indulgences without guilt. This balance can help you maintain a healthier relationship with food and reduce the risk of overindulgence when you "break" a strict diet. Consider the 80/20 rule, where 80% of your meals are balanced and nutritious, while 20% allow for flexibility and treats. This approach can help you stay on track without feeling restricted.

When making healthy eating choices, it's important to listen to your body and recognize its unique needs. What works for someone else might not work for you, so be open to adapting your diet to suit your lifestyle and preferences. The key is to find a sustainable approach that aligns with your goals and doesn't leave you feeling deprived.

In summary, making healthy eating choices without feeling deprived involves embracing flexibility, enjoying a variety of foods, and practicing mindful eating. By adopting this balanced approach, you can achieve a healthier lifestyle while still enjoying the foods you love. In the following chapters, we will explore additional strategies to help you maintain a sustainable and fulfilling approach to health and well-being.

CHAPTER SEVEN

Incorporating physical activity into your daily routine

Incorporating physical activity into your daily routine is a key component of any weight loss program. Regular exercise can help you burn calories, boost your metabolism, and build muscle mass. In addition to these physical benefits, regular exercise can also improve your mental health and mood, making it easier to stick to a weight loss plan over the long term.

There are many different ways to incorporate physical activity into your daily routine, and the best approach will depend on your personal preferences and fitness level. Some people prefer structured exercise programs, such as going to the gym or taking fitness classes, while others prefer more casual, unstructured activities like walking, biking, or hiking.

One popular way to begin incorporating physical activity into your daily routine is through a form of cardiovascular exercise.

Some examples include:

Running, jogging or walking on a treadmill

Riding a bike, either indoor or outdoor

Swimming, Dancing, Jumping rope, Participating in a sport like basketball or soccer.

These types of exercise can help you burn calories and boost your heart health. They also help in improving cardiovascular function, which will enable you to perform other forms of exercise more easily.

Another important aspect of weight loss is strength training. This includes activities such as lifting weights or using resistance bands. Strength training not only burns calories but also helps build muscle mass, which can increase your metabolism and make it easier to lose weight.

Another way to stay active is through daily activities such as house chores, standing and walking more often, and taking the stairs instead of the elevator.

It's important to set realistic goals for yourself. When starting a new exercise program, it's important to start slowly and gradually build up your activity level. It's also important to listen to your body and not push yourself too hard, too fast. It's better to start with short 20-minute sessions of exercise and gradually increase the duration and intensity of your workouts as you become more fit.

Incorporating physical activity into your daily routine is a great way to lose weight and improve your overall health and well-being. With a little bit of planning and determination, you can make exercise a regular part of your life, and reap the many benefits it has to offer.

Another way to make exercise a regular part of your daily routine is to find activities that you enjoy. When you find an activity that you enjoy, you're more likely to stick with it, which will increase your chances of success in your weight loss journey. There are many different types of activities to choose from, such as:

Yoga or Pilates, which can help to improve your flexibility, balance, and core strength.

Hiking, which can be a great way to get outdoors and enjoy nature while getting some exercise.

Team sports, such as basketball or soccer, can be a fun way to get some exercise and also improve social connections

Dancing is a fun way to stay active and get your heart rate up, many gyms offer dance-inspired classes like Zumba or Hip Hop

Outdoor activities like gardening or lawn mowing

Incorporating physical activity into your daily routine doesn't have to be an all-or-nothing proposition. It can be as simple as taking a brisk walk for 10-15 minutes during lunch, doing a quick workout at home before you start your day, or taking the stairs instead of the elevator. The key is to start small and build up gradually. As you become more fit and comfortable with your new routine, you can increase the duration and intensity of your workouts.

An important aspect of weight loss is consistency. It's essential to make exercise a regular part of your daily routine, rather than an occasional thing. It's also important to be patient with yourself. Weight loss is not always a linear process, and you may have ups and downs along the way. It's important to stick to your plan and not get discouraged if you don't see immediate results.

Incorporating physical activity into your daily routine is an excellent way to lose weight and improve your overall health and well-being. It's important to consult with a healthcare professional before starting a new exercise program, especially if you have any pre-existing medical condition or haven't been physically active in a while. The most important thing is to find activities that you enjoy and that you can commit to doing on a regular basis. With a little bit of planning and determination, you can make exercise a regular part of your life, and reap the many benefits it has to offer.

Let's take an example of a person named Sarah, who wants to lose weight and improve her overall health. Sarah has been sedentary for the most part of her life, and she has never been a fan of exercise. She decides to start incorporating physical activity into her daily routine as a step towards her weight loss goal.

Sarah starts by setting small, attainable goals for herself. She begins by taking a brisk walk for 10-15 minutes during her lunch break at work. She finds a nearby park, and she decides to walk around the park while enjoying her lunch. As she becomes more comfortable with this routine, she gradually increases the duration and intensity of her walks. She starts to walk for 20-25 minutes during lunch, and eventually, she starts to jog for short distances.

Sarah also starts to focus on strength training at home. She buys a set of dumbbells and starts doing bodyweight exercises like push-ups and squats. She starts with only a few repetitions, but as she becomes stronger, she increases the number of repetitions and the weight of the dumbbells. Sarah also finds an online yoga class that she can do in the comfort of her own home. She starts with a beginner class and gradually progresses to more advanced classes.

Sarah also starts to make small changes in her daily routine to increase her overall activity level. She takes the stairs instead of the elevator, walks to work instead of taking the bus, and she starts to do her own gardening and lawn mowing.

As Sarah consistently incorporates physical activity into her daily routine, she starts to see the results. She loses weight, feels more energized and healthier. She also starts to enjoy exercise and finds it as a way to relax and de-stress. She finds herself looking forward to her daily walks, yoga classes, and strength training sessions.

Sarah's example shows that it is possible to lose weight and improve your overall health by incorporating physical activity into your daily routine. It takes time, patience, and consistency, but with a little bit of planning and determination, you can make exercise a regular part of your life and achieve your weight loss goals.

Incorporating physical activity into your daily routine is essential for overall health and weight loss success. It offers benefits like improved cardiovascular health, enhanced mood, and increased metabolism. Consistency is key, so find ways to make exercise a regular and enjoyable part of your day.

To overcome common barriers like lack of time or motivation, consider breaking exercise into shorter sessions and exploring different types of activities to find what you enjoy. You can add physical activity to everyday tasks, like taking the stairs or walking the dog. Setting realistic goals and tracking progress can help you stay on track, and finding a workout buddy or fitness class can provide social support and accountability.

It's important to listen to your body to avoid overexertion and injury. Balance high-intensity workouts with lower-intensity activities like stretching or yoga. By incorporating these strategies, you can create a sustainable and enjoyable approach to physical activity that supports your health and weight loss.

CHAPTER EIGHT

Overcoming challenges and setbacks

Losing weight can be a challenging and difficult process, and setbacks and obstacles are a normal part of the journey. However, with the right mindset and approach, you can overcome these challenges and achieve your weight loss goals. Here are some strategies for overcoming challenges and setbacks when trying to lose weight:

Set realistic goals: One of the biggest reasons why people experience setbacks in their weight loss journey is because they set unrealistic goals for themselves. It's important to set achievable and realistic goals for yourself, whether it be losing a certain amount of weight in a specific time frame, or simply making healthier choices in your diet and exercise routine. By setting realistic goals, you'll be more likely to stay motivated and on track.

Track your progress: Keeping track of your progress is an important aspect of weight loss. By regularly monitoring your weight, measurements, and food intake, you'll be able to see how far you've come and identify areas where you can improve. Tracking your progress can also help you stay motivated and on track, especially when you see yourself making progress.

Be patient: Losing weight takes time, and it's important to be patient with yourself. Don't get discouraged if you don't see immediate results. Remember that weight loss is a journey and setbacks are a normal part of the process. Instead of focusing on the setbacks, focus on the progress you've made and keep working towards your goals.

Get support: Losing weight can be tough, especially when you're doing it alone. Surround yourself with supportive friends and family members who will encourage and motivate you. Joining a support group or working with a weight loss coach can also be helpful.

Identify and address triggers: One of the major setback in weight loss journey is often having triggers, that makes us fall back in our previous eating habits. Identify the specific situations or emotions that trigger you to overeat or make unhealthy food choices. Once you know your triggers, you can develop strategies to avoid or manage them.

Don't give up: Setbacks are a normal part of the weight loss journey, but they don't have to be the end of the road. Don't give up on yourself just because you experience a setback. Instead, use it as an opportunity to learn from your mistakes and make the necessary adjustments to get back on track.

Make healthier choices: Oftentimes, people try to lose weight by drastically cutting down on their food intake or drastically increasing their exercise routine, which can be both difficult to stick to, and bad for your health. Instead, try to make healthier choices in your diet, such as eating more fruits and vegetables, and in your exercise routine, such as incorporating more low-impact activities. These small, incremental changes will be more sustainable in the long term and help you achieve your weight loss goals.

Practice self-compassion: It's easy to get hard on yourself when you experience setbacks or obstacles in your weight loss journey. But it's important to remember that everyone has slip-ups and setbacks. Instead of being harsh on yourself, practice self-compassion. Remind yourself that you're doing the best you can and be kind to yourself. Self-compassion can help to boost your motivation and resilience, which are essential for overcoming challenges and setbacks in your weight loss journey.

Refocus on your motivation: Sometimes, it can be easy to lose sight of your motivation when you're facing obstacles in your weight loss journey. It can be helpful to take a step back and remind yourself of why you started this journey in the first place. Whether it was to improve your health, feel better in your body, or have more energy, refocusing on your motivation can help to reignite your passion and drive to achieve your goals.

Don't make it all or nothing: Often people feel like a setback is the end of the weight loss journey. But remember that weight loss is a journey, not a destination, and the setbacks are a natural part of the process. Don't give in to all or nothing thinking. Recognize that it's ok to slip up sometimes, and don't let a setback keep you from getting back on track.

Don't compare yourself to others: One of the most challenging parts of losing weight is not comparing yourself to others. Social media, friends, and other people's progress can make us feel inadequate and it can be detrimental to our own progress. Keep in mind that everyone's journey is different and what works for someone else may not work for you. Keep the focus on yourself, your progress, and your goals.

Find other ways to cope: Sometimes, weight gain or setbacks in weight loss can stem from emotional or mental health issues such as stress, anxiety, or depression. Finding other ways to cope with these issues can help to support weight loss. This can include mindfulness practices, therapy, or other forms of self-care.

Using the fictional character Sarah as an example, let's explore some strategies for overcoming challenges and setbacks in her weight loss journey.

Sarah has set a goal to lose 20 pounds in the next three months. However, she quickly realizes that sticking to a strict diet and exercise plan is harder than she thought.

She finds herself struggling with cravings and temptations, and often finds herself indulging in her favorite high-calorie foods. As a result, she is not seeing the progress she had hoped for.

Set realistic goals: Sarah recognizes that losing 20 pounds in three months may have been an unrealistic goal. Instead, she revises her goal to a more achievable target of losing one pound a week, which will still give her the desired outcome within her timeframe.

Track her progress: Sarah starts tracking her food intake, weight, and measurements, which helps her to see how far she has come and identify areas where she can improve. She also uses a food and exercise journal to keep herself accountable for the choices she makes.

Be patient: Sarah knows that losing weight takes time and that setbacks are a normal part of the process. She reminds herself to be patient and not to get discouraged if she doesn't see immediate results.

SUMMARY

The No-Diet Diet" offers a comprehensive and transformative approach to health and wellness by rejecting the traditional concept of dieting. It emphasizes the importance of building a sustainable lifestyle that fosters a positive relationship with food, body image, and overall well-being.

Key points explored in the book often include:

- Breaking Free from Diet Culture: It advocates for breaking away from rigid diet plans, restrictive eating patterns, and the pressure to conform to societal beauty standards. This theme highlights how diet culture can contribute to unhealthy behaviors, stress, and negative self-perception.

- Mindful Eating Practices: The book encourages mindfulness in eating, suggesting that paying attention to hunger and fullness cues can lead to a healthier relationship with food. It promotes savoring meals, eating slowly, and enjoying a variety of foods without guilt.

- Balanced Nutrition and Moderation: Instead of promoting strict rules, the book typically advocates for a balanced approach to nutrition. This involves eating a variety of foods, incorporating different food groups, and understanding that no food should be completely off-limits. Moderation and flexibility are key concepts.

- Emotional and Psychological Well-being: A central theme in the book is addressing the emotional factors that can influence eating habits. It explores how stress, emotional triggers, and psychological patterns can impact food choices and offers strategies for managing these influences in a healthy way.

- Building Long-term Habits: The focus is on creating sustainable, long-term habits that support physical and mental health. This approach contrasts with quick-fix diets or extreme weight loss methods, promoting a lifestyle that is enjoyable and realistic.

"The No-Diet Diet" ultimately guides readers toward a more holistic perspective on health, encouraging them to embrace their bodies, cultivate a positive mindset, and prioritize well-being over the pressure to conform to specific body ideals or dietary trends.

NOTES

NOTES

NOTES